T0154020

Overcoming Thyroid Symptoms

Overcoming Thyroid Symptoms

Your Personal Guide to Renewal, Re-Calibration & Loving Your Life

Vannette Keast

NEW YORK

LONDON • NASHVILLE • MELBOURNE • VANCOUVER

Overcoming Thyroid Symptoms

Your Personal Guide to Renewal, Re-Calibration & Loving Your Life

Published in New York, New York, by Morgan James Publishing in partnership with Difference Press. Morgan James is a trademark of Morgan James, LLC.
www.MorganJamesPublishing.com

ISBN 9781642798654 paperback
ISBN 9781642798661 eBook
ISBN 9781642798678 audio
Library of Congress Control Number: 2019952262

Cover Design Concept: Jennifer Stimson

Cover Design: Christopher Kirk www.GFSstudio.com

Interior Design: Chris Treccani www.3dogcreative.net

Editor: Moriah Howell

Book Coaching: The Author Incubator

Author Photo: Jennifer George Photography

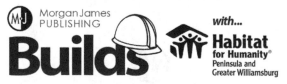

Morgan James is a proud partner of Habitat for Humanity Peninsula and Greater Williamsburg. Partners in building since 2006.

Get involved today! Visit
MorganJamesPublishing.com/giving-back

In Loving Memory
of
Dr. Lyle Smith.
1939-2019

My mentor and friend. As a Chiropractor he helped
many of us in my community to be relieved of pain for
over 60 years. As a human BE-ing, Lyle was a champion
to many, was kind, had a huge heart and he will be
forever remembered as an inspiration and an example of
'having made a difference'. He was to the profession of
Chiropractic, as Mother Teresa was to her religious order
and church.

Thank YOU Lyle for having been!

Disclaimer

The information, ideas, and recommendations contained in this book are not intended as a substitute for medical advice or treatment.

Please read this important note in reference to the many suggestions here-in for therapies and the consumption of specific foods, remedies and supplements.

1. Results will vary from individual to individual because we each have differing needs and a unique ability to respond both physically and emotionally. For any therapy or treatment to be effective, it needs to be tailored to each person to some degree. We are all unique in our ability to change and make the appropriate choices to act.

2. Information and statements within this written work have been made for the purpose of heart-felt caring and education. None of the information presented is intended to replace the advice of a doctor or medical professional. I am not a medical doctor. I do not dispense, nor do I provide medical advice, prescribe, or diagnose. In my writing and my work, I analyze and make meaningful and purpose-filled suggestions. My views are not intended to be a substitute for conventional medical services.

On a personal note, I have great respect for every professional who is devoted to quality medical care. I invite you to take personal responsibility for your own care to ensure you always receive the very best support and to make wise decisions to take good care of yourself. There is no one more important!

Table of Contents

Foreword   xi

Part 1:   **Background & Theory**   **1**

Chapter One: Introduction – Destiny & Change   3

Chapter Two: What Is the Thyroid &
Its Role in the Body?   19

Chapter Three: The Global Epidemic   29

Chapter Four: Causes of Thyroid Disease
& Imbalance   43

Chapter Five: Choosing a Whole System
Approach to Healing   61

Part 2:   **The Thyroid CARE Program**   **65**

Chapter Six: CARE - Cleansing & Clearing   69

Chapter Seven: CARE – Acceptance, Alignment
                   & Balanced Movement   91
Chapter Eight: CARE – Replenishing &
                   Nourishing   97
Chapter Nine: CARE – Evolution &
                   Recalibration   107
To Our Future   113

Acknowledgments   119
With Heartfelt Gratitude   119
Thank You!   125
About the Author   127

Foreword

I met Vannette in 2003 in a spiritual breakfast group that I had belonged to. Vannette was just joining our group that morning. The group leader introduced her and told us about her intuitive healing gifts.

At the end of that first breakfast meeting, Vannette and I introduced ourselves to each other. She reached out her hands to greet me and, as we held hands, she asked me if she could tell me what she saw about my health. Curiously, I agreed. She proceeded to accurately tell me about the health symptoms I had been experiencing – symptoms no one else in the room knew. She then told me that she knew how to help me heal. In that moment, I felt tears entering my eyes. In those first few moments with Vannette, there was something that felt like a knowing of each other – a recognition and trust that ran deep. I trusted that she had some answers and I had an inkling that we might fast become friends.

For the previous two or three years, I had suffered with insomnia and extreme fatigue. By each afternoon it was a struggle to think, and even speak, because I had so much brain fog. It was interfering with my work and my relationship. Only a month before my encounter with Vannette, I had made a firm decision that no matter what, I was going to find the source of this debilitating fatigue. I was very certain I could work out the way to heal myself. I had also reached out for help in prayer.

When I'd set out on the journey to heal my fatigue, it was difficult to even find a doctor that would cooperate with me. The doctors I encountered seemed only marginally interested in spending the time to help me solve this health puzzle. I suspected I might have an issue with my thyroid, but after the first doctor tested my thyroid, and those results showed thyroid function within a normal range, he was unwilling to do more tests. I recall him saying that it was too expensive to run all the other possible tests to find out what else might be causing my condition.

Finally, I did find a doctor that was open and willing to take charge in helping me solve this puzzle. He ran every blood and urine test that made sense so that we could find out what was going on. It felt good that I was finally getting some scientific data about what might be causing the fatigue. From these test results, there were more clues, but it remained that we could not pinpoint or conclude a cause. As a next step, the doctor booked me for a sleep study, and a barium digestive tract test. This is where I was when I started my program with Vannette; these medical tests were booked, but not yet done.

Within a month of working with Vannette, I called my doctor and canceled all of my appointments. I was sleeping much better, my brain fog had lifted, and I had a lot more energy. This "chronic fatigue" was lifting. I was starting to feel like my old self again. I could, once again, do my work with energy and confidence. Vannette had been the answer to my prayers for healing.

The work I did with Vannette was very similar to the programs she outlines in this book. I followed her customized program with commitment and devotion. I wanted to be well. Of primary importance was the cleansing that I did. This included physical cleanses as well as cleaning up the foods in my diet that were interfering with my absorption and energy. The custom program had me cutting out coffee, dairy, and wheat from my diet. That was not easy. Like most people, I loved my coffee and I had come to depend on it to function. Wheat-based food, like bread and pasta, were my comfort foods. Every day, under the program, I did the lemon/oil cleanse (found in this book). My program also included adding certain foods, vitamins, herbs, and minerals to my diet. I had a monthly session during which Vannette fine-tuned the supplements and cleanses to support each stage of my body returning to health.

At the same time that I had embarked on this physical healing journey, I began yet another in-depth cleanse and continued to clear my mind of limiting beliefs and emotions. Working with the mind turned out to be my own passion and gifting. I learned how to reprogram my subconscious mind with empowering new beliefs, and how to release stuck emotions and trauma. I also began coaching and teaching my own clients how to do this – supporting them in changing and healing their lives.

Vannette and I became fast friends and colleagues. A few years later, we shared a physical space in Calgary where Vannette would have her clinics one week of each month. She would work with her clients, and I would work with mine. In later years, we occasionally worked together with more "complex" cases, combining our gifts and intuitive capacities to help clients heal the core of their dis-ease. As you will read in this book, the true source of dis-ease will always be at the level of emotion and mind, but that is not always where the healing journey begins.

I have come to know Vannette as a powerful, compassionate healer and guide. She has a way of connecting with her clients that builds immediate trust. She tells it as she sees it, delivering her intuitive, angelic messages to her clients with empathy, compassion, and an authority that people trust. I have witnessed how she works with others, and how her clients have trusted their lives with her. She is a master at solving health puzzles that the medical system is either unable or unwilling to take on. The calling to unravel the mystery of increasing thyroid dysfunction, and how to resolve it, came to the right place. Vannette has the passion, the experience, and the gifting to receive and deliver this important, holistic thyroid health message to the world! If, in your own quest for healing, you have ended up here with Vannette, then, from my own experience, I assure you that you are in good, healing hands.

Many blessings,
J. Richard Schultz
WisdomWays
www.wisdomways.net

Part 1:

Background & Theory

Chapter One:

Introduction – Destiny & Change

For many years, I have watched as the thyroid gland has become a common concern. When I began work in the healing field, I observed that thyroid illness was a confusing condition because there was always so many other health upsets that appeared at the exact same time. Over time, however, with the help of my intuitive gift, I came to understand that these seemingly unrelated health upsets, appearing alongside thyroid symptoms, were not separate at all, but rather parts of the whole.

It is with a feeling of destiny that I share with you that I have become intimately aware of the connections between these various symptoms and how to interpret the message behind it all. I have come to the place of unraveling certain mysteries of health and this has helped me to support my clients in overcoming their thyroid symptoms. It is my intention that the information contained within this book will assist you in your process and journey to vibrant health, and to discovering your authentic voice.

WHO AM I TO BE SHARING THIS INFORMATION WITH YOU?

I am a Medical Intuitive and Emphatic Healer. Born with a heart to serve, I am continually in awe of this life, and aware of the great honour I have been given to be here now.

Mostly my experience of "reality" does not match with the consensus of what would be considered living a "normal" life. Let me give you a sense of some aspects of my world:

- I have full memory of choosing to come here. I was offered the assignment of this life and I agreed to it. An Old Soul, I am here by choice.

- I have always known realms beyond this physical reality and have "visions." Very often at the same time as I have visions, I hear "messages." Sometimes I only hear. The ability to receive information in this way is called "clairvoyance" and "clairaudience." As a child, as with all children who do not cognize beyond what is presented, I thought that this ability was common to everyone. My visions have always come in full colour and are always related to life and how I can be of assistance either directly with action or how my knowing allows me to BE a bright light of love and presence. In the visions I see people in many differing forms, places, and objects. The messages appear as a light, in an image of actual words, or a voice. The messages can be as simple as a word or two and oft as elaborate as a complete conversation. For example, the entire time I am writing this book, I have been supported by a "Guide" who is at this moment standing at my right side. He is cloaked in an indigo coloured, hooded robe. He has no visible face. I have come to know this "non-Earth BE-ing" as a representative from a group called, "The Hathors." He and his community are often with me. I have been shown that although I see him by himself often, he is always standing at the front of a collective of an infinite number of others like him. I am told that they are here to protect and care for humanity.

- I believe in Angels. They appear to me in gentle colours and though they do not speak, their presence, as is commonly understood, embodies protection, love, and encouragement.
- I have a council of Guides who are always available for me. They are a question away I say! These wise ones continually answer my questions and deliver clearly articulated messages.
- I can see the human body and its workings with the precision of an MRI scan.
- I have an innate understanding of metaphysics and the quantum field. I can see, feel and hear energy in all things. In all of life there is ebb and flow.
- I have an innate understanding of balance.

- I have a knowing of the energetic sequencing of love and how to translate the entirety of it into ''care'' for all and everything.
- For many years, I have identified as "multi-dimensional." I am continuously aware of worlds beyond this physical one in which you and I dwell. In these other worlds, life presents itself differently and simultaneously with this physical world. I consciously travel go back and forth between these worlds. For me, there is no veil separating the seen and unseen.

In the early days of sharing my gifts, after fully embracing the commitment to my purpose, it felt totally right and easy to trust that that both love and light would guide me in the correct direction. I came to travel only the paths that were illuminated. I would be nudged when I was to correct my course forward. As the richness of the silence expanded for me, I would listen, study, research, and show up where I was guided to be. As I took training and heard the many varied messages, I attained a mounting capacity to understand and harmonize with the wholeness that was body, mind, and spirit. I have come into an awareness of seeing, feeling, hearing, and knowing that we are all here to love life, and be loved by life.

WHAT IN THE WORLD IS HAPPENING?

In this time of rapid change, many speak of the palpable and nearly tangible sensation of life speeding up and of how the world around us is becoming increasingly unfamiliar. The pace of this acceleration is easily perceived by looking back over the last 100 years and noticing how our society has evolved. We have come so far in such a short time! We came from a reliance on the horse-drawn carriage to where now we travel freely with phenomenal speed by land, air and water. We have come through an industrial revolution to the development of nuclear power to a digital information age to where we are planning for the colonization of other planets in our solar system. Medical advancements have dramatically increased our life expectancy. Today, nearly every independent person in every western household owns a cell phone, a computer and a car. Advancements like these are happening at an increasing pace.

What of our future? 5G is upon us and artificial intelligence looms, whether we feel that we can trust these new technologies or not. Yes, lots and lots is happening!

We have much adjusting to do as we maneuver through the continual change everyone is watching unfold.

CHANGE IS

Change has always been a natural part of our human experience. However, the pace and volume of change that is occurring now is new to the human experience. This causes stress on the thyroid in several ways.

Firstly, change is generally unnerving to the basal nature of human beings. When it's fast, it can upset every aspect of our innate our balance. Uncertainty and distress can commonly lead to panic, causing some people to become depressed or anxious or even intermittently both. Because the thyroid gland is a regulator, intense emotion and sustained fear will always have a negative impact on it.

Secondly, we cannot easily opt-out of the diverse changes and transformations going on

in our world. Gone are the days when we could choose whether to have or reject technology; think of the common-place of the television, microwave or dishwasher. There was a time when we could choose whether we were going to upgrade – and when we made the choice, we would adopt the new item, complete with the learning curve that accompanied it. In former times, we believed that we were in control of the pace of how new things filtered into our daily life. In recent times, with so much unavoidable change, many feel powerless to stop "it," or to slow "it" down. This feeling of powerlessness too, directly affects every aspect of us and especially the thyroid gland.

Thirdly, we know that the pace and acceleration of change is not a temporary phenomenon, but an integral and permanent part of life in our current time. As a result of this, I find that many are feeling an intense "fear of the future". This too directly affects us all in every way and especially upsets the thyroid. Change IS happening everywhere.

- *The weather is changing:* Temperatures in some regions are colder, while in others it's hotter than anyone can remember. The seasons are not coming-and-going with the same familiar regularity. There seems to be an increase in the events of flooding, drought, mudslides, fires and even summer snowstorms. Day-to-day, whether we are looking to make a geographic move, plan for an outdoor wedding, or start a construction project, the weather can dominate planning.

- *The way we get news has changed:* Socially, we once relied on corporate news networks to tell us of the happenings of our times. It was television, radio, magazines and newspapers. Now, social media is considered the new norm and within minutes any message can be circulated the world over. As a result of this change and other factors, many of the smaller market and community media outlets that had been, have long been permanently closed.

- *Institutions are changing:* Many mainstream institutions that were central to our communities are needing to fully over-haul in an effort to reflect current expectations. Those that do not are failing. For example, many secrets and hidden practices are being exposed. I think of the Catholic Church and its many secrets that were once hidden away and are now out in the open. As many celebrate justice and transparency, others mourn the loss of innocence or of what 'was'.

- *Communities are changing:* Everywhere we live, work, play, and interact our communities have a new look and sound. We are now a collection of people comprised of multiple cultures, customs, and languages. Human migration and changing social norms have challenged us to accept more diversity than ever before. We are being asked to embrace differences like never before.

- *The consciousness of humanity is changing.* At the exact same time that some will roll up their sleeves to engage in the current turmoil and the societal unrest, there are just as many who reject every notion of a fight. These individuals believe in peace and will focus on making it central to daily living. Herein is one aspect of how we can see that society is intensely polarized. It seems to me personally that we are all in the same place of innately looking to equitably reconcile both differences and all injustice - and that we are just going about it differently.

- *The face of nature is in change:* The Earth we ALL call home is different than it was. How so? A few include: 1) The tectonic plate activity and the extreme weather. Many areas on Earth can no longer support the traditional habitat due to the changes. This is causing life of all forms, plant, animal and human, to either move or disappear. 2) Human population encroachment. As we build and spread out to house and feed our growing numbers, natural habitats are permanently altered and even destroyed. 3) Pollution and toxins. Present everywhere, these are consumed by all of life on the planet. 4) Modern science. All modifications to the genetics of any life form will have an impact on both the overall terrain of nature and all other life forms. Yes, the balance of nature has changed and continues to change. Just how resilient are we all? The one thing we know for sure, is we who live on this planet are in this ALL together.

- *The cosmos is in change:* The sun is our single source of light and heat. All of life on this planet is directly dependent on it for survival. According to scientists, leading up to approximately 2012, there was a gradual and measurable change in the amount of solar flaring. Today, we are now fully in a time of reduced solar flares. Also, that this planet is traveling through a new stretch of space. A brand new place in our orbit and one where this civilization has never before journeyed. As a result, the entire surface of the Earth has been increasingly flooded with both a larger volume of radiation and varied new types of radiation. I see that it is this radiation and our reaction to these new varieties that is directly impacting the functionality of the thyroid gland. We are undeniably being called to adapt and to trust in a process that seemingly few have the awareness to describe. All of life on Earth is in need to do this consciously and unconsciously while having no expectation to control any aspect. It's happening equally to us all, for us all. Yes, we are to live today with the optimism that soon a new dawn will appear on the horizon. This is the essence of what is happening at this time.

CHANGE CAN TRIGGER A CYCLE OF GRIEF

When change happens, even positive change, there is always something lost. This loss commonly triggers grief. Grief is how human beings process loss. If the loss is monumental and intense, the emotions accompanying grief can shut down both our desire to communicate and our ability to speak. Often, our survival response to intense change is to shut down the movement or expression of emotion, and to deeply internalize everything. Emotions are meant to move: E-Motion is energy in motion. Shutting down or internalizing emotions and trauma, adversely affects our body, negatively impacts the thyroid, and plays a key role in altering its function.

Change challenges our existing beliefs, forcing us to adapt in order to survive. In these times of rapid, complex change, our entire BEing is being pressured to release what used to make sense, and to embrace the new. To accept these profound changes, our thyroid gland must constantly re-balance and align with these new physical and emotional states.

According to many modern-day thought leaders and teachers – those grounded in the work of conscious awareness and those who channel sentient beings - humanity is growing in compassion. We are thought to be entering into a phase of existence where the choice to have compassion will enhance us and is fueling the activation of our re-calibration. More and more, it is seen that many of us are choosing to live in peace and be grateful. Each time an authentically caring communication and action takes place anywhere on this planet, it affects the very fiber of our collective existence and it creates positive shifts that create a type of affect that benefits all of society. What we do and how we choose to BE in our daily lives, matters.

According to Kryon Book Thirteen titled, *The Re-calibration of Humanity*, we are in a slow and gradual transference to another level. I understand this text to mean that as we evolve and change, a renewal is happening. Could all of this be meaningfully intended to have us discover that we are each capable of focusing on what is of the highest and greatest of good? Can we finally let our differences fall away? As talked about by my childhood friend Lee Bussard in his book titled ''More Alike Than Different,'' indeed we are much more alike than different!

MY FRIEND DAVID

Recently, I visited a long-time friend who was in hospital. On a variety of medications, David had been plagued with one mystery illness after another for about 20 years. It all began after he was in a work-related accident that nearly took his life. He had had every symptom of thyroid illness, from hair loss and weight gain to heart palpitations. Now, in a severely weakened state, he shared that his heart was damaged so severely that it would no longer function independently of the machines beside him. The pacemaker, installed the previous year, could not help him. That day, he was in a lot of pain from the edema that had him swollen to nearly twice his normal weight. David was having a hard time breathing; he was in tears. He was scheduled to be tested the next day to see if he was a candidate for a heart transplant. Holding David's hand, running energy and praying, I could not help thinking that there was so much good this big-warmhearted man could be doing, were he not confined to his bed.

Later that evening, in the stillness of silence, I heard a familiar voice. It spoke clearly to instruct me that it was time *to speak out and speak up*. It told me that my time of working quietly was to end, and that I needed to reach a larger number of people who were just like my clients and my friend David. The voice assured me that all would organically reveal itself to me and that I was to write and speak as I am here now.

A NOTE OF RECOMMENDATION

Most recently, I see that there is an ever-increasing presence of light in our world. It is a brightness that is inside each if us and is everywhere. Will this light illuminate the path forward for us all? I invite you to be curious, ask questions and listen to your heart and connect to your own intuitive guidance. There is nothing like the power of a question to guide us into the ever-expanding truth.

Chapter Two:

What Is the Thyroid & Its Role in the Body?

So, what is the thyroid? Where is it located? What does it do?

The thyroid is a gland that is part of our body's endocrine system. The endocrine system is a collection of glands that produce and secrete hormones that regulate the activity of cells and organs in the body. According to the current understanding of our human biology, these hormones mainly regulate metabolism (the physical and chemical processes of the body), growth and development, tissue function, sexual function, reproduction, sleep, and mood, among other things.

Designated as a master gland, the thyroid is one of the most important. It produces the hormones thyroxine (T4), triiodothyronine (T3) which are regulated by the pituitary gland release of the thyroid stimulating hormone (TSH). T3 and T4 hormones influence every cell, tissue, and organ in your body. Your thyroid regulates the rate at which your body produces energy that comes directly from the nutrients you consume and the oxygen taken in. It provides an aspect of balance or regulation for overall energy and cellular function. I see it as a harmonizer in that a healthy thyroid will maintain a constant and natural rhythm as it dictates homeostasis.

Every bodily function relies to some extent on a healthy, fully functioning thyroid gland. For example, the functions of kidney rhythm, fluid level presence, heart rhythm and strength, libido, fertility and reproductive health, as well as brain function and memory, are a few of the vital functions that are governed by the thyroid gland. The thyroid gland is also connected to gastrointestinal function, adrenal hormone metabolism, blood-sugar levels, stomach acid and bile production, liver and gallbladder function, and all the detoxification processes. A dysfunctional thyroid, therefore, can be a significant contributor to the manifestation of almost any malfunction in the body system - this truth is often overlooked in the standard diagnosis of disease.

THYROID GLAND INFOGRAPHIC

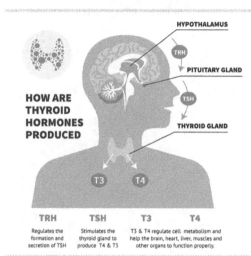

HOW ARE THYROID HORMONES PRODUCED

HYPOTHALAMUS

TRH

PITUITARY GLAND

TSH

THYROID GLAND

T3 T4

TRH	TSH	T3	T4
Regulates the formation and secretion of TSH	Stimulates the thyroid gland to produce T4 & T3	T3 & T4 regulate cell metabolism and help the brain, heart, liver, muscles and other organs to function properly.	

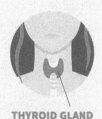

THYROID GLAND
THE THYROID GLAND IS A BUTTERFLY-SHAPED ORGAN LOCATED IN THE BASE OF YOUR NECK

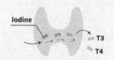

Iodine

T3
T4

THYROID GLAND TAKES IODINE, AND CONVERT IT INTO:
- thyroxine (T4)
- triiodothyronine (T3)

THE THYROID'S HORMONES REGULATE VITAL BODY FUNCTIONS, INCLUDING:

HEART RATE   BODY TEMPERATURE   MUSCLE STRENGTH  BODY WEIGHT

MENSTRUAL CYCLES   NERVOUS SYSTEMS CHOLESTEROL LEVELS   BREATHING

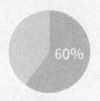

60%

UP TO 60 PERCENT OF THOSE WITH THYROID DISEASE ARE UNAWARE OF THEIR CONDITION

Diagram 2a

If you were to take a look at pictures of the thyroid gland in a modern-day biology textbook, you would notice that it is located at the base of the neck and it appears to be shaped like a butterfly. However, according to my intuitive sight, I have always had a view of the thyroid as being in the shape of a five-petal flower. Energetically, I see it functionally comprised of three main lobes (petals) that are vibrant and active, and two lobes (petals) that were dormant, until recently. These two sleeping and silent lobes are now stirring with energy and have begun to wake up. Yes, they are gaining in vitality and are ''powering up.'' I see this as hugely meaningful and a real change that is affecting our whole body.

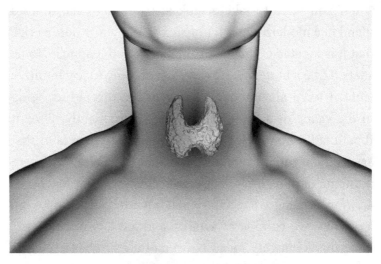

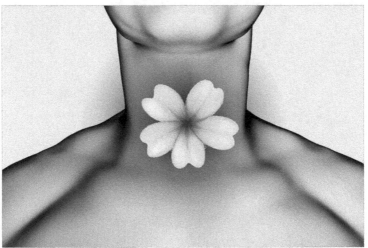

In my journey of understanding the thyroid gland, I have been shown that each of the lobes have had very important and individual functions.

- The first lobe plays a key role in harmonizing brain function – balancing the likes of serotonin and dopamine, making for clear-thinking, problem solving and intellect in general. In this, the first lobe influences mental health, memory, and the ability to concentrate and learn.
- The second of the lobes has a direct role in kidney function – the kidneys filter the blood to remove waste, control the balance and rhythm of fluid and adjust the blood for mineral and electrolyte balance. Edema and inflammation are two common physical discomforts that I see resulting from kidney disharmony and inefficiency and a reduction in the vibrancy of the second lobe.
- The third lobe affects heart function – its ability to beat rhythmically, effectively and efficiently. A non-negotiable factor in sustaining life, many an episode of heart failure or mystery heart illnesses coincide with various symptoms of thyroid gland upset.

- The two newly active lobes. Though their precise role is yet to be shown to me in its exact form, I am certain of their significance and how our entire human expression is to be affected. Considering that the thyroid is currently operating at about 60% of its capacity and expression, how will we be at 100% capacity? I see that as we evolve over these coming years, many aspects of our presence will become enhanced. This is the recalibration I speak of. To me, this feels like we, as a collective, have arrived at an open doorway to a bright and spectacular new world! Everyone everywhere is being affected. I have been shown that many of the current symptoms of thyroid gland upset are the growing pains in this phase of evolutionary adjustment. Furthermore, our yet-to-be born will eventually arrive with all five lobes of the thyroid gland functioning in complete harmony.

At the same time as I had begun to notice these new vibrations and the light frequency shift in the thyroid, I became aware that the colour of the thyroid energy had shifted dramatically. It had always been blue – a beautiful Mediterranean Sea shade of blue. Although this sea blue colour remains in that area of the throat as aligned with the fifth Chakra, the thyroid gland itself has become the colour of TEAL. This now stable appearance of the colour teal, synonymous with the thyroid gland, is to me a confirmation of an energetic alignment with the heart. Yes, this beautiful flower is blossoming and expanding its influence on the body as it gains in its expressed brilliance! We are becoming greater and more than we have been.

Chapter Three:

The Global Epidemic

Thyroid disease and dysfunction are on the increase globally. Some would describe it as an epidemic, and trusted professionals tell us that the reason for the rapid increase of thyroid issues is largely unknown. An additional concern for them is that thyroid dysfunction is difficult to diagnose due to the complexity and wide variety of symptoms that can be associated with it.

Another reason thyroid dysfunction is very often not observed as problematic is that specific symptoms are often treated as a standalone. With the task – diagnosis and treatment – in check, it can be seen as being resolved with no clinical reason for a deeper investigation into root causes. For example, a symptom of hypothyroid is depression, and instead of diagnosing the thyroid as problematic and supporting thyroid function directly to remedy the illness, an antidepressant drug is most often prescribed.

Here are just a few indicators of this global thyroid epidemic and its impact:

- On a global scale, it is now estimated that a staggering 200 million people have problems with their thyroid glands.
- Already the most common endocrine cancer, the incidence of thyroid cancer has dramatically increased worldwide in the past few decades. It is increasing at a higher rate than any other type of cancer.
- The incidence of Hashimoto's thyroiditis (HT), considered to be a chronic autoimmune disease related to the thyroid, has increased in the past two decades, paralleling the trend of increased thyroid cancer. Hashimoto's is considered the most universal autoimmune disease and it's estimated

to currently affect approximately thirty million women.

- It is estimated that at least sixty percent of thyroid disorders remain undiagnosed. It is predicted that nearly half of all women, and a quarter of all men, in the USA will die with evidence of an inflamed thyroid.

SYMPTOMS OF THYROID DYSFUNCTION

The most common symptoms of an impaired thyroid gland are extreme fatigue, insomnia, intermittent or constant extremes of feeling cold and numbness, brain fog, depression, anxiety, constipation, hair thinning and loss, weight gain, general aches and pains, and goiter. Other symptoms include diabetes, the inability to conceive, infertility, menstrual upsets (from irregularity to debilitating pain), menopausal symptoms, heart palpitations, chest pain, gout, edema, kidney area pain in the mid to lower back, kidney and bladder infection, viral infection, rheumatoid arthritis, autoimmune disease, and cancer. Each of the symptoms in this list can be an illness on its own and, left unchecked, each has the potential of becoming problematic.

It seems to me that the time has come for us to put real effort into determining the basal cause of illness and to understand that nearly every illness experienced today involves some aspect of a struggling thyroid gland. Because thyroid function is not yet widely understood, it is up to each of us to be informed, pro-active and personally accountable. Whether you or your loved ones are experiencing thyroid symptoms or are seemingly symptom-free, it is wise to choose to be pro-active and engage in habits of daily thyroid care.

DIFFICULTY IN DETERMINING ABSOLUTE DYSFUNCTION

Because there are many and varied symptoms of thyroid upset, and that each major symptom in itself has the potential of being diagnosed as a specific illness, it is extremely difficult for the modern mainstream diagnostic system to make an absolute determination. This alone, in my opinion, is the cause of misdirection and confusion. Additionally, on any given day, many a health test can conclude differing results from the previous testing. Why? Because in every moment all aspects of life have influence and impact – basic health, emotional state, the foods chosen and compatibility to that food, stress and environmental conditions are among the most common factors.

The traditional, medical way of testing for thyroid gland efficacy is through blood and saliva tests. Western medical professionals look for evidence in the blood, while Naturopaths and Integrative professionals commonly look at the saliva or a comparison of both blood and saliva. In alternative medicine, I, like many of my colleagues, use a range of other testing systems and approaches. These includes energetic testing, bio-resonance testing, reading body signs, muscle testing, listening and truly knowing the client to understand their perspective and to have collaboration whenever possible.

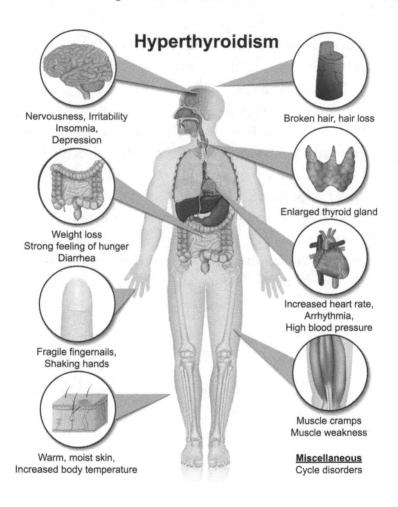

Hyperthyroidism

Nervousness, Irritability
Insomnia,
Depression

Broken hair, hair loss

Enlarged thyroid gland

Weight loss
Strong feeling of hunger
Diarrhea

Increased heart rate,
Arrhythmia,
High blood pressure

Fragile fingernails,
Shaking hands

Muscle cramps
Muscle weakness

Warm, moist skin,
Increased body temperature

Miscellaneous
Cycle disorders

Hyperthyroidism: Excessive production of thyroid hormones

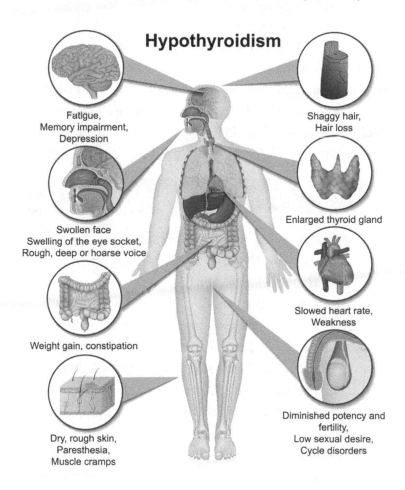

Hypothyroidism

Fatigue,
Memory impairment,
Depression

Swollen face
Swelling of the eye socket,
Rough, deep or hoarse voice

Weight gain, constipation

Dry, rough skin,
Paresthesia,
Muscle cramps

Shaggy hair,
Hair loss

Enlarged thyroid gland

Slowed heart rate,
Weakness

Diminished potency and
fertility,
Low sexual desire,
Cycle disorders

Hypothyroidism: Not enough production of thyroid hormones

Case Stories of My Clients

The following are stories of three of my clients whose varied symptoms of thyroid imbalance are indicative of the complexity of this dysfunction. More examples and details will appear later in this work when I delve into the CARE Program and other customized healing processes.

CASE STORY – MARY:

Mary had all the early signs of thyroid imbalance in her late teens. By 21 she was getting intermittent chest discomfort and pain, her hairline was thinning and the cold sore activity that had first appeared when she was twelve, had been getting worse. She was now 26 and having trouble sleeping, had menses irregularity, was often very cold and had severe constipation. Weight gain had become rapid and she was frightened by how the chest pain and arrhythmia were now waking her in the night. Having undertaken all the routine medical tests a few times, she was at a loss because her results were always the same - a little low but within normal range.

The following is the treatment process she has been following.

- Mary commenced with each of the cleanses mentioned in this book, did a four-day intensive liver cleanse and followed an enema routine. On a daily basis, she now starts and ends her day with warm lemon water, consumes supplements that support positive intestinal flora and has continued to do a light cleanse for one week every month. Her plan is to do more intensive cleansing once or twice annually. She understands the importance of keeping the elimination system clearing.

- As her diet was already quite clean, we made the tweaks nutritionally to include consuming foods that naturally contain iodine and nutrients that helped her specifically improve her digestion and the natural ability to eliminate.

- Her enhanced supplement intake included magnesium, zinc, lysine, selenium, vitamins E, A, D, C, B in addition to products that included both Cayenne, Turmeric, and Garlic.

- In addition, Mary agreed to take time each day to be in stillness. From the calm she found she was able to reach deeper states of healing. She did this through meditations and in spending extended time in nature settings – some days standing by a tree on her lunch break or going for a walk on the grass, other days spending time by a stream at her community park. She also did regular sessions on the Crystal Bed & Amethyst Bio Mat therapy system that I use in my clinic.

- The other therapies included: Topical use of iodine and products that supported her entire endocrine system and several homeopathic remedies intended to support the weakening of the virus believed to be responsible for cold sores and many other maladies.

- Mary is stable at this stage. Her weight gain stopped immediately after beginning the protocols and the variety of changes recommended; she continues to lose weight slowly. Her outbreaks are currently lessening in both event and intensity, the heart palpitations are much fewer and much less intense when they arise, she has new hair growth, and is mostly sleeping through the night and waking rested.

CASE STORY – SUE:

Sue, a 50-year-old businesswoman, had a visible protrusion from her throat (goiter), had gained 70 pounds over the past 20 months, suffered from insomnia, was exhausted all the time and was experiencing disabling brain fog. Though it was obvious that her throat area was enlarged, her test results showed that the thyroid function to be in normal range. Although she began to feel better within a few weeks of having made a number of changes, it took nearly six months for the obvious lump that was showing to slowly shrink. The goiter has now nearly disappeared though Sue continues to feel some strain when she swallows.

What healing program or process worked for Sue?

- Her diet was changed to clear and clean her digestive and elimination systems. Many changes were essential as she had many cravings and coped with life using a number of foods that were not compatible.

- She completed three months of a cleanse protocol. At the same time she was applying topical iodine and consumed Kombu, Selenium, Bee Pollen, Iron, vitamins E, A,

D, C, B, Magnesium and Curcumin. Sue also responded well to homeopathic remedies intended to generally enhance her immune system and to weaken the significant viral and bacterial signatures that were present.

An added observation was that every time Sue went off the food recommendations and made an effort to wean off what was being suggested in the protocol we had created for her, the goiter would visibly increase in size. Based on this, my recommendation to Sue was that she would now need to go deeper into herself and her beliefs to further unlock the additional requirements. It was obvious that what we were doing was successfully managing the condition, however the root cause was not being addressed. Sue needed even more self-care than what she had agreed to do.

Steve, a 41-year-old dairy farmer, who also tested as normal for thyroid, came to me with intense joint and back pain, severe insomnia, and exhaustion. He also had a severe skin rash, extreme constipation and the most upsetting of his symptoms was constant gout in three of the toes on his right foot. I found that Steve was highly reactive to milk products, and many other foods he loved, all of which he was regularly consuming. Reluctantly, because he struggled with the concept of not consuming the primary product that his farm produced, and hated change, Steve decided to commit to just one protocol. He said he felt his options were very limited as he had sought every official medical council available to him – that it was worth trying just one protocol.

We began with a focus on substantially changing his diet. He applied topical iodine, consume a volume of both kelp and vitamin C in addition to homeopathic remedies.

Within a week, almost every symptom was substantially improved – the rash was almost gone and his right foot no longer throbbed making the pain finally manageable. After 2 months and several adjustments to his initial protocol, his gout had disappeared, the skin rash had vanished, and his overall pain was minimal.

Like Sue, when Steve would miss his supplements or cheat a little to consume foods not recommended for him, the reaction would be immediate and upsetting. He shared with me recently that he felt like a new man and that he and his family were growing closer once again.

Chapter Four:

Causes of Thyroid Disease & Imbalance

L ike every disease, though the bottom line seems to determine what has gone awry, the source of the upset and the exact cause is always unique to that person. Though a huge number of people today will have thyroid gland dysfunction, the severity of it will vary greatly. Why is that? Because though we humans are a lot alike, we are also quite unlike anyone else. Our experience and perceptions are seldom viewed as the same as our neighbor's. The way I see it, the path to discovering how to create and sustain healing starts with being honest with self and can then include a daily practice of self-care coupled with finding peace in BE-ing. Who am I? What do I want? What do I truly need? What is the causal chain or source of each upset? Also, to be considered in the mix are factors such as: the environment, beliefs, emotional upset and trauma, genetic tendency, immune system vibrancy, stress response and the overall body, mind and spirit harmony. It is from this place that meaningful change can happen.

Getting to the source can be complex and difficult to determine because it is often obscure. I have found that to have lasting success with healing of any kind, one must consider both care for the immediate minute and for the whole. By whole, I am referring to physical, mental, emotional, and spiritual. By immediate minute, I mean to focus on relieving immediate discomfort, pain and weakness. For example, a client named Joe came to me with a chronic shingles outbreak. It had been going on and off for nearly six months and of everything he had been doing to get it to stop, nothing was helping. Supporting Joe to get relief from the extreme discomfort was paramount. However, this needed be done alongside identifying how to weaken the viral grip and to find the source of the upset. It turned out that the physical symptoms arrived within a week following a major automobile accident. This was his second accident in two years and in the first his best friend was killed. In this case, the combination of both physical and emotional trauma were the conditions that weakened the body, allowing the virus to gain in vitality. Hence, the base cause of his shingles outbreak was trauma.

Today's medical model has a primary focus on physical symptoms. It is as if the premise of modern medicine is to hold the view that suffering and human tragedy is exclusively physical, mechanistic, and biochemical. As this medical model struggles to remedy chronic issues with medication and surgery, many many people suffer. With alternative-to-western practices, though we too look at the physical symptoms, our consideration goes far beyond any surface appearance to the whole system where the root cause can always be found. Once root cause and the causal chain is determined, then the body is encouraged to unwind from the stress. Healing is a matter of commitment to care and individualized support. Take the time, you are soooo worth it!

CAUSES OF THYROID ILLNESS – THE PHYSICAL, ENVIRONMENTAL, EMOTIONAL & ENERGETIC

Viruses, Other Invaders & the Immune System

The virus: 100 times smaller than a single bacterium, these complex non-living (as we know life to be) organisms are currently very difficult to find and to identify. With thousands of known viruses, it is quite easy to imagine that we are all both positively and negatively affected by their existence. Those we commonly see as a bother on a regular basis are responsible for warts, cold sores, the common cold and flu, along with outbreaks like Shingles. However, the nastiest known viruses are at work draining our life force without visible evidence of their presence. Considered quietly destructive, they are many and varied and include the likes of Epstein-Barr, Herpes, and Hepatitis.

Because modern medicine often does not look to find the base cause of illness, and instead treats the symptom, the average person has little awareness beyond trusting in the determination of a name for their condition and receiving a prescription. In my work, I have found that in every case I have worked with involving thyroid disruption, there is evidence of at least one immune draining presence - a virus, parasite or bacteria. In some cases, all these types of invaders are present to some degree. The CARE program in part two of this book has been created to outline ways to strengthen your immune system and to reduce the influence of harmful viruses that degenerate wellness and directly have impact on thyroid health.

Genetics

We have all noticed family tendencies toward specific illnesses and types of disease. Many of my clients will tell me about their family pattern and be resigned that this too is their fate. One of my clients, Jenny, stated that every member on her mother's side had been on thyroid medication since she could remember, and that her father's mother and his three sisters were all on this same medication too. She was sure there was nothing that could be done to prevent her approaching demise. As many people, she believed that what has always been, always will be.

One of the first teachers and leaders to speak of how our genetics need not rule our destiny is Dr. Bruce Lipton. In his book, *The Biology of Belief*, Dr. Lipton explains that, although we may have inherited a gene for a certain disease or a non-pleasant physical tendency or weakness, the genes themselves do not turn on or off based on our genetic programming. According to his research and view, the genetic expression is influenced or triggered by how we think and believe about our environment and our world. In other words, Dr. Lipton teaches that we can take the wheel and we can drive our genetic expression through reprogramming our subconscious mind to create health. It is really and truly our choice alone that creates our reality. We are not victim to the circumstance of our lives. As we refuse to accept limitations and illness, we can install positive and healthy concepts that support us to manifest states of health and empowerment. Furthermore, that with self-love, love of all and the goal of peace inside us and outside us, we can turn on the genes that help us each to create the best version of self that we can be!

As Lee Carroll, who channels Kryon, once told me personally, "Illness is part of the old paradigm." He has referenced repeatedly for decades that the human body was created to live for hundreds of years. Recently, he is quoted as having said nine hundred to be exact. I, too, wonder what it will mean for me personally and for our society, I am told yet again to ''get out of my own way''. Yes, like many of us, I am a work in progress. As I take-in all that I hear and am shown, I take comfort in Dr. Lipton's voice on his YouTube channel and in his teachings. I invite you to take a personal inventory and determine where you too are standing in your own way and not living your true potential?

Dental

A whole, complete body approach to dentistry involves the knowledge that our teeth and oral health is an important barometer of overall health. Each tooth is a direct indicator of the wellness state of a very specific organ, gland, and at times a system function. Our body is comprised of a type of invisible wiring system that carries our vital life-force along twelve energy pathways known as meridians. Specific to the thyroid gland, there are eight individual teeth that align directly with the function of the thyroid gland. These teeth are called the Bicuspid. There are two on the upper and lower of both sides of the mouth. If these teeth have decay, take a physical blow or are deprived of nutrition or circulation, the energy flow along that meridian will be impaired. This will in turn affect the ability of the thyroid gland to function with the ease that was intended. The opposite can also happen – if the thyroid is compromised, the teeth too can be affected. The working of our human body is truly exquisite! I see that its magnificence is akin to that of a symphony. If even one instrument is not properly tuned or the timing is temporarily lost, the performance will be negatively affected.

Not recognized commonly at this time in our way of life, this knowledge comes from a Chinese model that is more than 5,000 years old. Yes, I am certain that dental health is an important consideration when determining the physical causal chain and when seeking the path to implementing whole healing.

Radiation & Solar Storms

According to solar physicists, until approximately 7years ago, our planet had been in a place of orbit in the Milky Way where solar flaring and radiation was consistently fluctuating but mostly constant within a predictable range. Since 2012, we have been travelling through a place that our current civilization has not experienced before. As dependent as always on the sun for light and heat, our location as it is now, is resulting in both reduced solar flaring and evidence of an increase in both the intensity of radiation and in the types. American science journalist, Deborah Byrd, asserts that this pattern has continued from 2012 to present time and that it is expected to continue on into the foreseeable future.

What does this mean? It is known that changes in solar flaring can increase the occurrence of geomagnetic storms here on Earth. These storms cause disruptions to our power grid and electrical systems and we are vastly dependent on the grid for all aspects of modern living such as electricity, communication, satellite, and GPS. I suggest that, if our technology is troubled by events stemming from our cosmos, then we humans are hugely affected too.

What does this really mean for you and I? With the entirety of our atmosphere containing both new types of and an overall increased volume of radiation, we are being affected every day. Further, that as our thyroid gland is especially sensitive to radiation, we cannot ignore that everyone, everywhere is being impacted.

Could this be a matter of human survival or fodder for our growth? I believe that this is our destiny and that everything happening has been meant for us. Our body is quite simply, in an adaptation process. As our thyroid gland makes its adjustments to regulate homeostasis, our expression is meant to become varied. It is renewing and recalibrating.

Emotional & Energetic

Emotions

A natural response to anything and everything that is considered unfamiliar, or perceived as threatening, is fear. Our instinctual reaction to fear is to either freeze like a deer facing oncoming headlights or to escape like a squirrel that disappears with lightening speed up a tree. Internationally acclaimed horse-trainer and author, Pat Parelli, references the horse as a prey animal. Horses are highly reactive to any "thing" suddenly introduced as unfamiliar – a person or thing or an unanticipated action. To a horse, unfamiliarity is usually perceived as dangerous, and can give them cause to look to escape. In the hierarchy of the animal kingdom, humans have much in common with those classified as a prey animal.

Our management of any fear is central to our health. Defined in the book *A Course in Miracles,* fear is opposite to universal love. On page twelve of this brilliant classic you can find the passage that has made all the difference in my own life: "Perfect love casts out fear. If fear exists, then there is not perfect love." I interpret this to mean that as darkness and light cannot be present in any one moment - so too does the presence of love eliminate fear. Love and fear are opposites. It is like when a flashlight beams into the night, all the the darkness ceases.

Healing cannot happen in an environment where fear exists. With so many varied reasons to be overwhelmed and afraid in our daily lives now, today, it is essential that we each know how to secure our personal peace. Nothing is more important than to have a supportive practice as a tool. Will you BE a vibrant example of One who both chooses peace and IS peace? I see that we are to rise above our instinct around fear – we are to challenge our biology and to mindfully manifest certainty, confidence and strength. As our thyroid works to support us, we are charged to become both the best we can BE and to be examples for all the others around us.

Energetic - The Chakra & Blockages

According to eastern-based spirituality and many modern healing models, the human body can be viewed through a systematic configuration known as Chakras. There are seven primary Chakras and, like acupuncture meridians are vibrant unseen energy pathways, the Chakras are non-visible energy centers. Each one of the Chakras is associated with both a specific colour and with a unique frequency and vibration. They are believed to regulate many physical, emotional and spiritual processes. In this system, trauma and self-limiting beliefs or stuck emotions are known to block a Chakra of its expression and its essential flow of energy or chi.

The fifth Chakra is located immediately at the base of the neck at the throat and the physical place of the thyroid gland. According to this system, this energy center is associated with expression, communication, speech, and emotion. It is believed that the following types of common current day upsets have a negative impact on the function of both this Chakra and the thyroid gland:

- When a person has gone through a sustained upset or trauma where they were unable, not allowed, or chose not to speak or express themselves.
- When a person has been powerless to speak up for themselves or for a loved one.
- When those from whom they seek approval, do not respect or honour their spoken word or opinions.

Commonly, each of these experiences will result in a sense of helplessness that triggers a high level of stress and ultimately the desire to hide or escape. People who have had this experience can go on to create a lifestyle that results in needs not being met, which in turn result in energetic restriction or emotional implosion on the fifth chakra. Over time, holding onto traumatic stories and the emotions associated with them further affects the physical gland. The result is that by restricting or pushing the thyroid gland off course, it is unable to properly regulate the streaming of energy and its ability to do its physical job.

To survive upsetting and traumatic life experiences, we often apply logic to make sense of the upset or to justify what has happened. Arising directly from this logic and/or any justification, the subconscious will imprint the experience. This can become a blockage to health. Known as a mind virus, it is important to your health that you release these blockages, so that more peace can prevail. The types of beliefs that will impact thyroid health are among the following.

- People don't listen to me, hear me, or understand me.
- What I have to say is not important.
- Nobody cares about my opinion. My expression is not welcome or respected.
- Expressing myself gets me in trouble – best not to do that.

- It is not safe to express myself or to speak out.

According to my guidance, every client with thyroid pathology needs to delve into this realm of beliefs to seek out the root cause. Belief change work is about taking steps to release the stuck emotions, downgrade trauma, change or reprogram the old patterns and correct the erroneous stories that no longer serve a person in a positive way.

Environmental Toxins

Most of us have been exposed to a multiplicity of unhealthy chemicals and toxins. It's impossible to avoid exposure to the toxicity that is everywhere, in every form: city, town, and even countryside. While there is no toxin that is good, the following toxins are commonly present in modern living and have been noted as especially upsetting to the thyroid gland: pesticides (agriculture); BPA (an industrial chemical that has been used to make certain plastics); bromine (an additive to oils and liquids); perchlorate (anti-static agent); PFC (found in boxes and mattresses); fluoride (toothpaste, urban water treatment); and preservatives in food.

Fluoride is one toxin that is particularly harmful to the thyroid gland. The thyroid gland is known to be comprised of the most fluoride-sensitive tissues in the human body. Referenced as a toxic industrial waste product in the 2013 documentary film created by Dr. David Kennedy called <u>Fluoride Gate - An American Tragedy</u>, exposure is repeatedly cited as a major contributing factor to the increasingly common medical findings of thyroid illness. Fluoride, according to Dr. Joseph Mercola, undeniably interferes with the functioning of the thyroid gland. He is an outspoken advocate for the removal of it from widespread use.

How does fluoride upset the thyroid gland? Its presence has been found to increase the concentration of certain thyroid hormones while decreasing the production of others. It is known to mimic TSH (thyroid-stimulating hormone) and irreparably damage it, which interferes with homeostasis. In addition, it prevents efficient iodide transport causing iodine to be unavailable and starve the thyroid of its ability to function, repair and regenerate. Fluoride also blocks enzymes that balance the thyroid glandular secretions (for example deiodinases are necessary to convert T4 into T3) and in turn can cause many functional upsets including intelligent brain function, kidney capacity and the proper beating of the heart. It has been stated that prolonged fluoride exposure will cause the thyroid gland to become fully suppressed.

Many scientists and health professionals recommend avoiding fluoride completely and/or to maintain a minimal exposure. It's further interesting that, as recent as 40 years ago, fluoride exposure was the medically sanctioned treatment for an overactive thyroid gland (hyperthyroidism).

Physical Trauma

Physical trauma of any kind will always affect the entirety of the person. However, when a blow to the head or throat happens there will be some form of structural shifting and also the probability of thyroid function interference. Physical upsets such as that experienced in an automobile accident or a fall or being struck are among those I see as especially having impact on the thyroid gland. Often an injury of this kind can trigger illness related to thyroid function.

In effective self care, physical and hands-on therapies are important. Touch and feeling "cared for" is essential to human existence. The kinds of therapies I recommend include: Chiropractic, physiotherapy, acupuncture, laser therapy and massage therapy. Additionally, energy healing work is also very effective. Among those that I practice and am familiar with are: both in-person hands-on healing and at-distance-healing, crystals and treatment systems like a Crystal Bed and an Amethyst Bio Matt.

Chapter Five:

Choosing a Whole System Approach to Healing

Imagine the innate intelligence that it takes to organize and coordinate thirty-seven trillion cells of the human body to act as one whole system. Imagine the electrical and biochemical communication that must be occurring in every moment between these cells to move and act as one.

The human body has evolved over hundreds of thousands of years into a truly magnificent organism that supports our human consciousness for this incredible human experience on planet Earth.

I know that this vastly intelligent organism we call the human body has within it the blueprint and intelligence to create perfect health. Given the right conditions, the human body knows how to balance and restore itself in every way. The body, which completely regenerates and renews all its cells about every 7 years, knows how to be well. But if this is true, why is there disease?

It is claimed that, upon his deathbed, Louis Pasteur (1822-1895) said, *"The microbe is nothing. The terrain is everything."* In this statement, Pasteur was essentially saying that focusing on the microbes (bacteria, viruses, fungi) that were invading the body as a cause of disease was not the best focus (*it is nothing*). Instead, the environment (terrain), or the environmental conditions inside and outside the body, were greater determinants of health or illness. In other words, "fighting germs" was the wrong battle, or an incomplete one.

Originating from Pasteur's original views on fighting disease, our current medical and pharmaceutical model is still focused on the microbe rather than the terrain. The western medical thinking is also a left-brain, mechanistic model that views the body as a machine made up of parts and pieces, rather than a whole system of inter-relating parts working together and compensating for any imbalances. In a parts-based, mechanistic worldview, medicine tries to find the broken parts and fix or replace them. This is a narrow view of health, and while it works well for acute problems like a broken leg, it is limited in supporting and transforming the whole system of the body, mind, and spirit toward its innate state of well-being.

So what is meant by "terrain"? And what is optimal? How do we create the ideal conditions for the intelligence of the human body to find its way back to optimal health and balance?

In my healing practice and my holistic CARE system outlined next, you will notice that I do consider the microbes that can be involved in thyroid dysfunction. However, rather than focus on attacking a virus or bacteria, I have found that it is better to support and strengthen the immune system, and take good care of the environment or terrain, so that the body can do what it does best. The CARE system focuses on creating optimal conditions for the body; enabling it to use its own innate intelligence, such as immune function, to restore optimal health and balance. When the environment or terrain is healthy and supportive of the body, healing can happen quite naturally.

In the CARE system, the terrain or conditions include the inner and outer physical conditions that the body is exposed to, and it includes the conditions of the mind such as unresolved trauma, stuck emotions, and limiting beliefs and thoughts about health. Specifically, it asks what toxins (physical, emotional, and mental) need to be cleansed or released, and inquires about what nutrients and energy need to be added to the system for the body to thrive. As the body moves toward health, the CARE system is about appreciating, adjusting, balancing, and re-calibrating to support the body at each stage of its healing process. For example, in the first stages, you might need to focus at the physical level such as cleansing your body of toxins so that your body can absorb the nutrients it needs for renewal. Then, once you have more physical energy, you can move on to do the deep emotional work of the mind to transform the root causes of the dysfunction. This is a process. This is patiently and lovingly taking CARE of the whole of you so that you inwardly and outwardly can thrive in your experience of life.

Part 2:

The Thyroid CARE Program

The purpose of the following chapters is to share that there is no better time than now to *see, feel, hear, and know* that we can choose to take independent, positive actions to be healthy, to self-heal, and to have a healthy, functioning thyroid gland.

There is a path to health. We can make the most of all the elements that have impact on us, including from our universe, the planet, technology, society, community, and our self-perceptions. We can choose to have a much better experience in this life. No matter how tired, weak, ill, discouraged, or anxious you may feel, I know you can take a step in the right direction. You can do it! By taking even one small step, you will begin traveling a path that is sure to lead you to much more health, vitality, and happiness.

CHOOSING TO HEAL

Did you know that the very first step to doing anything meaningful is always a decision? We often forget that every journey anywhere always begins by looking at our various choices and deciding. Your choice may be about whether to continue on in the direction you have been going, and the actions you have been taking, or to embrace a new path and new actions that present themselves. There is always choice.

Perhaps you are part of a family that has had generation after generation of life-limiting health and illness. Maybe your mother, grandmother, uncle, or brother have thyroid illness. Perhaps you notice similar illness among your friends and within your community. If, or when, you notice these things, do you feel resignation that these deficiencies are inevitable and will happen to nearly everyone you care about? Could you choose to believe in yourself and your own strength? Could you believe that you are innately designed to be healthy, and that you *can* trust in your ability to *be* so?

Choice. There will always be a choice. The decisions we come to will reflect our own sense of self-worth and what we believe is possible for us. What does it mean to be truly worth it? What would it be like to feel so worthy of health, love, and abundance that you break rank with the familiar and the limiting habits and beliefs, and forge ahead with conviction and determination to face a future filled with the unfamiliar? To be clear, I am not projecting right or wrong here. My remarks here are to illuminate the crossroad before us all and to shine a light on the choices. Which direction will you travel at this intersection of your life?

I will beckon you to walk the way of being open-to-newness – to the unfamiliar. I ask you to take-to-heart the real possibility that you have been inherently designed to consciously own your power and take responsibility for self-healing and renewal. I invite you to be present and trust that, once you make a decision for health and abundance, a brightly lit path will appear to guide you. Consider to BE truly open to receive that radiating love. Are you ready to fall in love with yourself, and your life, anew?

In the next chapters, I will outline a holistic approach to thyroid CARE that speaks to all levels of your being and addresses healing to your core:

- **C**leansing & Clearing.
- **A**ppreciating, Aligning, & Balancing.
- **R**eplenishing & Nourishing.
- **E**volving & Re-calibrating.

Chapter Six:

CARE - Cleansing & Clearing

In our modern society, chemical compounds, negative microbes, and viruses are everywhere and it's impossible to prevent them from having an impact on our health. Realistically, awareness of the possibility of their presence is helpful, but there is no doubt that dealing with toxicity or pathology is a complex process. If you feel that this is true for your thyroid condition, and you feel you need assistance, I implore you to seek out the appropriate professional care and feel free to contact my office so that I can be a further source of assistance.

I refer to cleansing and detoxifying as being akin to spring cleaning your home after months of snow, freezing temperatures, and a preference for hibernation. This is a common ritual for most people, no matter the climate. However, it is especially customary for those of us who live in the northern regions of the world. In the months of cold temperature, the fireplace is stoked, and the pantry will be full. When the warmth of spring finally returns, everyone is keen to freshen up cozy inside spaces.

In the spirit of "out-with-the-old and in-with-the-new," our precious bodies have such a need to cleanse and be clear. The ability of the bodies to do intestinal purging is essential to the health overall, and especially the thyroid gland. The ascending colon, located on the right side of our abdomen, is the place of tiny receptor sites that directly feed the regenerative processes of the thyroid gland. If the ascending colon is not clear, but rather congested and sluggish, then this lining of matter is preventing the thyroid gland from receiving the nutrients necessary to its healthy function. It's very important to your thyroid gland that the intestinal walls are continually clearing and that positive bacteria (gut and intestinal) have a supportive environment.

In this cleansing and clearing section of the CARE program, consideration will be given to ways to cleanse your colon, and your entire body, your environment, your emotions, and your mind. Let's clean up and let go of all those things that cause stress, block your energy, and that you no longer have need for.

PHYSICAL CLEANSING – BODY AND ENVIRONMENT

Body

As outlined in the last chapter, in our current day environment, we are exposed to multiple toxins that are man-made and unnatural as well as natural toxins that we would not normally be exposed to. Our amazing bodies, as advanced as they are in maintaining health and balance, have not evolved under these conditions and therefore are often incapable of adequately releasing or compensating for these harmful elements. Therefore, we need to help our bodies detoxify on a regular basis.

For safe and effective detoxification processes that can be added into your regular daily schedules, I encourage all ages to routinely participate in effective cleanses. The use of effective cleanses are essential to minimizing or removing the impact of the toxins listed and many more harmful toxins. Cleanses are also helpful with encouraging the entire elimination systems to operate at peak efficiency. Following are the actual cleanse systems that I use personally and have been recommending for intermittent use to others for many years. They cleanse, detoxify, and clear.

Cleanse One

Each morning – or morning and night – on an empty stomach, after brushing your teeth and tongue, consume a *drink* comprised of eight to twelve ounces of warm/hot water with the juice of half an organic lemon or lime added to the water. In the morning, wait for a minimum of 30 minutes after this drink before eating breakfast.

Note: If your teeth are free of amalgam fillings, consider doing an "oil pull" before drinking the lemon drink. An oil pull is done by placing a minimum of one tablespoon of a healthy oil (such as organic coconut oil) in your mouth, then swishing it around for at least 10 minutes before spitting it all out and thoroughly rinsing your mouth.

Cleanse Two

Each morning, on an empty stomach, first thing after brushing your teeth and tongue, consume a *drink* of eight to twelve ounces of warm/hot water complete with the juice of half of a raw organic lemon or lime. (You can also do the oil pull before this, if it is applicable to you). Wait a minimum of 15 minutes, and then consume the following:

Detox Pudding:

Combine the following and mix into boiling-hot water:

- 1 Tablespoon flax seed meal
- 1 Tablespoon psyllium hull
- A pinch of *Insan* bamboo salt or raw sea salt
- 1 Tablespoon chia seed
- An herb such as Milk Thistle or Slippery Elm that will give attention to the liver or bowel depending on the individual's focus
- Optional: Additions to this mixture are activated charcoal and bentonite clay at 1-2 teaspoons of each
- Mix this combination gently and regularly for a minimum of 15 minutes. It can be glutinous if it is not properly created – add enough hot water as needed to ensure that it combines with an even, fluid consistency.

- Once cooled, consume it through a large diameter straw.
- Follow this with additional water and brush your teeth.
- Wait 30 minutes before consuming food.

NOTE: Are you an individual with a strong "gag" reflex? Are you texture sensitive? Your taste-buds are ultra-sensitive? This intake may not be an option for you. If you are attracted to trying it however, know that the entire process could be placed into capsules. It is essential to consume a very large amount of water.

Cleanse Three

Before your evening meal, or as a snack by itself in the evening a few hours before bed, consume the following well-blended mixture:

- Half a whole raw organic lemon (rind, seed, juice, and all)
- 1 Tablespoon of a natural oil containing omega 3, 6, and 9 (I use hemp oil most often)
- 4 to 8 ounces of pure water
- If you need to have it less tart, add natural stevia to taste. No other type of sweetener should be added

because the drink needs to be alkaline- the addition of any sugar will create acidity.

All three of these cleanses can be done while carrying on with your normal daily routine. They can help both the liver and the bowel flush stagnation and undesirable residue.

Healing Tea

In addition to the above cleanses, to further support the healing and fortification of digestion during a cleanse, I recommend consuming the following enjoyable ginger-lemon tea. Most helpful to consume anytime mid-morning through to noon, it can be enjoyed any time of day. Combine the following into your favorite mug or a convenient to-go cup:

- Thinly sliced raw ginger, hot water, freshly squeezed lemon juice, stevia drops

Environmental

The cleansing of our unique environments is individual, based on lifestyle, occupation, and personal sensitivities.

- <u>Physical Home and Work</u> – First consider the area in which you live and work. A good start is as simple as choosing to minimize exposure to, and contact with, the chemicals and non-organic substances in your space. Be mindful to clear away the likes of aerosols and air-fresheners, perfumes, and chemical cleaning compounds.

- <u>Energetic Clearing</u> – Ensure your space is energetically free of impediments, and has every positive element present to encourage a healthy lifestyle. Energetic stagnation and unwanted energy signatures can be the cause of a heavy, unhappy-feeling space. Consider carrying out regular energetic clearings by doing rituals such as the following:
  - Walk from room to room with intention, or in prayer, and visualize that Divine light and love is filling-to-the-brim each room.
  - With loving intention, do one of the following: scatter sea salt, sprinkle essential oils, or burn dried sage or other herbs.

Consider the mindful process of applying the principles of Feng Shui to your home and office. I recommend Anita Adrain's book, *The Heart of Feng Shui...Simply Put* at www.fengshuisimplyput.com. Take into account these simple harmony-creating aspects:

- Live clutter-free for a free-flowing movement of energy and air.
- Open windows, blinds, and curtains every day to let in fresh air and sunshine.
- Decorate with vibrant, healthy plants.
- Diffuse essential oils.

Viruses and Microbes

The presence of viruses, bacteria, mycoplasma, and parasites are known to be the cause of many serious illnesses. These invaders can directly affect the healthy function of the thyroid gland. Epstein-Barr is an example of one virus of several known in the herpes family. Lyme disease is an example of one type of bacteria and a mycoplasma that is the smallest bacteria detected to date. Tapeworms and pinworms are two examples of millions of known parasites.

For my entire work, I have been highly aware of the pervasive and invasive nature of these invaders. As an intuitive, addressing their presence is always high in the priority sequence of the therapies I am guided to work. For complete healing, their presence must be either gone, or their effects minimized.

Personally, I was diagnosed and bedridden with mononucleosis twice before the age of twenty. Our family doctor made his determination based on symptoms only, because there existed no commonly available medical test to confirm it. Mononucleosis is known to be caused by the Epstein-Barr virus. It affects everyone from infants through to the aged. I have come to be certain that viruses, bacteria, and mycoplasma are one of the major factors to consider in the treating of every modern-day illnesses. Further, because they are always difficult to detect, due to their nature of "playing hide and seek," the impact of their presence is either not considered, or simply cannot be confirmed.

Here are some of the most powerful natural foods and compounds that can be used to support our bodies terrain in its ability to purge the invaders. Some are also known to weaken both viruses and microbes:

- **Foods, and Herbal Remedies, Compounds:** aloe vera gel and juice, asparagus, artichoke, berries (wild), celery, cilantro, coconut, garlic, ginger, onion, peppermint, raw honey, stevia, turmeric, colloidal silver, oil of oregano, oil of peppermint, black walnut, artemisia, olive leaf, echinacea, and cat's claw.

- **Homeopathic Remedies** by Physica Energetics: Mycelia Intrinsic, Viru-Tox, Mycoplasma-Tox, Mono-Tox.

Immunotherapy

Modern medical research is offering new ways for viruses and complex bacteria to be detected so they can be targeted for clearing. These types of therapies work at a cellular level to enhance an individual's immune response and to encourage die-off. I personally recommend a European based laboratory called the Research Genetics Cancer Center (RGCC). This international organization can be contacted in North America via the head office in Texas, USA.

Electromagnetic Frequency – EMF

Modern society is now almost completely dependent on electronic devices and wireless technology. These technologies emit EMF (electromagnetic frequencies), that have a dire affect on the body - particularly the thyroid gland is impacted upon due to its sensitive to this type of radiation. Common sources of EMF radiation include WiFi, cell phones, computers, televisions, home appliances and security systems.

It is unlikely that human health will be unaffected by the technological advances coming our way in 5G wireless connectivity. My suggestion is that, while most of us will not or cannot unplug, we can make every effort to unplug regularly and take time to go off-the-grid. In this way, it may be possible to minimize the effects of EMF and the other abhorrent frequencies present in our modern lives. The uncertainty of the effects of future electronic exposure is all the more reason to make serious choices in self-care. The following are examples of actions and practices that can be adopted with ease and effectiveness:

1. **Have a bath.** Soak in water that contains natural minerals and salts such as finely ground raw sea salt and/or Epsom salts, along with your favorite essential oil. I suggest not only to cleanse your body in this water, but to have an extended soak – for the length of time it takes to fully relax. It's also important to lie down in the water, at least up to the top of your neck, and to often submerse your

head. In this way, the thyroid gland is sure to be directly nurtured.

2. **Adorn yourself.** Wear jewelry made with natural materials like stones, wood, gemstones and lab-grown gems. They are alive and they are supportive because of their vibration in addition to their ability to accept our programming. Important that you find what works for you. For me, wood is one my personal favorites. I wear a ring that is hand-made from a wood scrap. And another daily favorite is either earrings or a pendant from the collection of Kate King, a Canadian jewelry artist. The most powerful for me is the white sapphire and both the Paraiba and the indigo.

3. **Take walks in nature.** Walk among the trees, or alongside a natural water source, and make a conscious effort to breathe deeply. Walk barefoot on the soil, sand, grass, or snow; wade into a stream. Be surrounded by nature. Relax in the sounds and the sense of it all.

4. **Meditate.** In whatever fashion you know to find your stillness, go in and BE silent and BE in the silence. From the calmness, I encourage you to be open to receive all that the Divine will provide to

assist you. This can be done when in a stationary place and it can be done equally effectively while moving. I totally enjoy the practices of both Tai Chi and Qi Gong. Some days what I find the most helpful is to go for a mindful and silent walk around the neighborhood or down a country road.

Specific to the thyroid gland? When in that calmness, imagine connecting with the energy or feeling the thyroid location at the base of the neck. Imagine that area infused with a teal-coloured light and lovingly hug it. I always see my thyroid gland as the blue-green five petal flower.

5. **Move the Lymphatic System**. In the design of our body, is the system of lymph channels and nodes that are called-upon (above any other single function) to carry impurities out of the body. The challenge this system faces is that there is no pump to move its contents along. Therefore, we need to assist the lymph action by daily choosing to be physically active. I recommend that one of the ways to ensure it is efficient is to be active each day by way of walking briskly, running, jumping, and/ or bouncing. Additionally, certain treatments and

tools can enhance the effectiveness of lymphatic action. These include far-infrared saunas and bio-Mats, ion detox therapies, lymphatic-release massages, and exercising in a heated, steamed studio as in the Bikram style of yoga.

Emotions

On an emotional level, it is best to make every effort to BE in peace and harmony, and to communicate in peace with everyone you interact or share space with. At work and at home, unresolved upsets will create an undesirable field. Even the slightest hint of tension is a negative presence.

How can something long-over-and-done be released or altered so that it no longer negatively impacts a person? There are specialized processes that can be done to do exactly that. Dr. Bruce Lipton's book, *The Biology of Belief,* expands on this subject. The method I use and have been using for years is the brainchild of a friend and colleague. He and I have worked with hundreds of individuals who sought to accept change and deep-reaching healing. Called *Wisdom One*, it is a ceremonial-based process that involves a high-level of intuition and observation. It is designed in such a way that an individual is supported to re-frame, downgrade, and forgive, a past upset or trauma. Through this process, limiting beliefs are reprogrammed, and stuck emotions and trauma are released. It is an experience that leads to healthier perspectives and to wisdom.

Mind

Our mind is known to play tricks on us. It can take us on a journey of ups and downs, rounds and rounds, leaving us dizzy – and all the while we've not even left our chair. Phew! I'd rather have the mind play the part of a dear friend who is a conveyor of useful information and wisdom. So how do we get the mind working for us rather than against us? How do we use it so it is supporting the caring and healing of our thyroid gland?

An exercise for you. Start by being quiet and centered in a place where you will be uninterrupted for a time of this engagement.

First step. Be mindful of the intention to be healthy, whole, and complete. Engage all your senses in this process and manifest what its like in your mind's eye: (a) feel how that feels in a tangible way/ is it smooth or fluffy? cool or warm? (b) smell it, (c) taste it, (d) see it (e) hear it. Assign a colour to your creation.

Second step. Believe in what you have created and make the decision that you are healthy, whole and complete. Apply that colour to your thyroid and all your body.

Breath it in and love what you lovingly created. Enjoy fully this perfect place and space that you created for you!

The power of your mind is well demonstrated in the work of the two brilliant teachers, Dr. Ryke Hamer and Dr. Michael Lincoln. They are similar in their unique perspectives on health and healing.

Dr. Ryke Hamer. According to Dr. Ryke Hamer, the founder of German New Medicine (GNM), all disease is the result of the mind's conscious awareness of a specific and significant trauma that has been viewed as not avoidable or not resolvable. Every isolating conflict shock is said to create an imprint upon the psyche that is translated to the brain, and if unresolved it goes on to have impact on the corresponding organ. This potential dysfunction or an imbalance with that organ, gland or functionality can result in disease.

Over the course of his career, Dr. Hamer was able to prove his theories by doing actual brain scans on his patients. In the case of the thyroid gland dysfunction, his text references serious conflict about "not being fast enough." His text suggests that each person would have his or her own personal version of how a situation or upset became a trauma, the conclusion would always be similar, according to Dr. Hamer. According to GNM, the basis of dysfunction of the thyroid gland would generally be fear of not being fast enough to do or be something that was desired, or fast enough to avoid an impending disaster.

The following are case stories of my clients that support the GNM theory.

1. **Fear of not being fast enough to avoid the collapse of the familiarity of their life.** *My client John was well aware that his partner had been unhappy for some time. Try as he might, nothing he did and did not do prevented the arguments and her seemingly erratic behavior. They had gone to counseling; he had even asked her to come and see me for counseling. Then, one day when he came home from work, she was gone. In the collapse that he went through, unable to make sense of it all, his thyroid gland went completely off-line. Along with John's physical healing journey, we worked to support him in all ways while he sorted through the loss. In the end, he was able to re-frame his story so he could forgive both himself and his lost love.*

2. **Deep regret and upset that they lost out because of being hesitant to speak about being in love with their chosen partner.** *Joy worked in a law office with a firm policy that employees were not to be involved outside of the office. She and James advised each other on almost every client case they worked on; for nearly 5 years they had lunch together almost every day. When she shared with him that she was looking for another office to join so that they could have the option to move their friendship further, he shared that he had recently become engaged. In her total shock, she was angry with herself and with James. She felt regret, and she perceived she had been betrayed. Joy had already been working with me in a general prevention posture and was shocked when nearly overnight she had full-on symptoms of thyroid upset. Because she was immediately supported to both release the emotional upset and to feed the struggling thyroid gland, she stabilized quickly. In the end, she took a position with a new law office and moved on, coming to embrace the blessings in this new chapter of her life.*

Dr. Michael Lincoln: According to Dr. Michael Lincoln, author of *Messages from the Body*, thyroid problems occur as a result of continual and repeated experiences of deeply troubling rejection. This glandular pattern of dysfunction would occur only after there was sustained suffering and deep emotional upset which would result in what he terms as a "failure to flourish" condition that is akin to the well-known Freudian condition of "fixation'" or, according to GNM, "maturity-stop." According to Dr. Lincoln, this person may then be actively in "victim mode."

In my work, I have watched success and miracles happen when a person is willing to recognize they are impacted by a wall of beliefs that are the result of a story that no longer serves them in moving forward with their present life. When they make the choice to walk through that wall, change their mind, and re-frame their perception with new and helpful concepts, the shifts are always profound. For some, choosing to forgive and embrace new concepts is a reasonably quick process while for others, where there has been repeated trauma, a longer process may be necessary. In the case of repeated trauma, I offer to start with the recovery process by doing a guided meditative process that I call Journeying. This process is performed with my client in a highly relaxed and quiet state. This process requires in-person presence. Over a duration of sixty to ninety minutes together, we work through a guided process that honors the person's requirement to receive answers. In it, we will visit the Akashic Record and be shown how to safely access and uncover the key to renewal.

Chapter Seven:

CARE – Acceptance, Alignment & Balanced Movement

Acceptance is the complete agreement to take in whatever spontaneously shows up in our life, and both fully experience the value that it is or has and appreciate it. Resistance is the opposite. I feel that real acceptance is the alignment with a natural forward flow of life and always results in peace. In my findings, peace is an essential requirement for healing.

My client, Calinda, came to me with a diagnosis of an autoimmune disorder. At first, she was hesitant to do anything outside the realm of her medication. She was afraid because she'd been so very physically ill. But her instincts told her that there was more that she could do. At 32-years-old with a 5-year-old child, she was struggling daily with the use of her hands; her mobility was becoming increasingly limited. She was cold all the time, loosing hair in handfuls each day and was gradually losing both weight and muscle. Motivated to have more physical ease, Calinda longed to remain active with her son.

I was convinced that we needed to go deeply into the cause of all her symptoms, and the cause of why she came here to be traveling this road to this disability. She initially made some progress in both vitality and circulation by way of a protocol designed to feed her physical body and to reduce her stress response. However, it was in working lovingly with her fears and beliefs that we began to see more rapid progress in her healing. It was with Calinda's acceptance to look at, and re-frame, what she believed to be unrelated experiences, that she began to allow the energetic shifts to really happen. Calinda is now not only playing daily with her son, she also plays and coaches soccer 9 months of the year.

I have no doubt that whatever appears in your life, it is there to help you understand how to BE or do your journey differently. Thyroid illness is always about trauma related to the suppression of voice and personal expression. With acceptance and tools, the life lesson that is before you can be understood and a course correct made possible. Our time here on Earth is precious and, with acceptance, one can make excellent use of the time we have.

PHYSICAL ALIGNMENT

Another consideration is structural alignment. If your neck, head, or shoulders are not properly in place, or there is pinching or subluxation, the thyroid gland can either be outside its proper place or out-of-sync with its natural rhythm. This will affect the thyroid's ability to do its job. How easily can this happen? It can happen from everyday poor posture, the result of stress, sleep position, falling and bumping the head or neck or taking a blow. Because there is no regular pain we associate with the thyroid, we are unaware of the upset around the physical location of it. My personal way of managing my life, to stay on top of being bumped about and physically stressed, is to make time for chiropractic adjustments and massage therapy. I recommend that everyone receive regular body work.

BALANCED MOVEMENT

Every healthy organ, gland, cell, and muscle is continually in motion and has its own rhythm. This makes sense when we think about the lungs or heart but all organs and glands are equally as active. When any function has its free flow interfered with or halted, the change in its function is almost immediate. Stagnation and toxicity will soon be factors in the region. Hence, I wish to make the point that movement is essential to the healing of any aspect of our body, mind, or spirit. Without movement, there can be no flushing and replenishing action. No matter your choice of activities like running, power-walking, jumping (especially on a trampoline), dancing, and swimming – movement helps with the essential free flow of all energetic aspects.

I have chosen one specific practice of yoga to exemplify how intentional movement, combined with mindfulness, has been long used to encourage healing. Bikram Yoga is a practice comprised of a sequence of twenty-six postures. It is performed inside a studio heated to approximately forty degrees Celsius, with a humidity of around forty percent. This duplicates the environment in India where this practice originated. Bikram Yoga evokes movement in both posture and in the lymphatic system. It is undeniably effective at stimulating meaningful and targeted movement while also assisting the body in detoxification.

Specific to the thyroid gland? According to Adam Chipiuk of Studio X in Edmonton, Alberta, of the iconic twenty-six postures and Bikram poses, those that feature pressing the chin down toward the chest are especially caring for the thyroid function. These are known as "compression poses". As part of my personal enjoyment of the Bikram practice, I include positive affirmations and a mind focus on healing intentions while doing this intense and rejuvenating moving meditation.

THROAT MEDITATION – HEAL THE THYROID

I have already mentioned using meditation and positive self-talk as a way to calm the mind, gain awareness, and reduce fear. Here is a meditation that I invite you to do regularly to support your personal overall wellness and to help your thyroid to function optimally.

- Step 1 – Prepare.

  Loosen your head and neck by doing neck rolls of a complete 180 degrees in both directions. Do a minimum of 8 in each direction, followed by the same number of movements in a figure eight (the infinity symbol).

- Step 2 – Sit erect or lie down for maximum comfort. Use pillows to support your posture. Hold your hands with palms open and relaxed.
- Step 3 – Straighten your spine, drop the shoulders, and tuck your chin slightly to create a neutral hanging position.
- Step 4 – Bring to mind the colour teal. Imagine seeing an orb in that colour. Close your eyes with the vision of the teal coloured orb and imagine that it is peacefully present in your physical throat area. Intend that it would float over and around your thyroid and feel like it is lovingly hugging you and your thyroid. *Note that you may even feel a vibration in your throat and thyroid region.*
- Step 6 – Continue for as long as your time allows, or as is desired.

Chapter Eight:

CARE – Replenishing & Nourishing

PHYSICAL REPLENISHMENT

I recall watching an interview with His Holiness, the Dalai Lama. He was asked, "What is the one thing commonly required by everyone and everything everywhere?"

He said, "Love, of course."

Afterward, he laughed and laughed. When he stopped the body jiggling from the joy, he added, "And almost as much, is laughter." To love and be loved is as vital to life as is the air we breathe. Laughter has long been called the best medicine. No matter what path brought you to this place and this time in your life and health, the manifesting of these two basics are non-negotiable essentials of life.

Love. It always begins with a love of self and includes all aspects of caring for yourself, with having a nourishing physical environment and personal space, along with all the best bits of community and peace. The importance of laughter begins with one's ability to laugh at one's self. It progresses to finding humor in all of life. Though laughing in itself physically exercises the throat and the thyroid gland, the sound of people laughing together is the very warmest. Laughter is one of the most beautiful uses of our voice.

Personally, I need physical touch to feel nurtured. To me there is almost nothing better than a cozy hug. What is it that you need to feel physically replenished and whole? Find it, dear One and ensure you always have it. You and your thyroid are depending on it.

NOURISHMENT FOR YOUR THYROID

The thyroid gland itself is quite simple to feed. Caring for it is all about recognizing it as a single, vital presence with special, sacred energy. The thyroid has the need to consume specific nutrients, to expel waste and invaders, and to be loved and appreciated. Here's how to easily and joyfully apply the best care.

Nutrients

The essential nutrients for optimal thyroid health are selenium, B12, iron, zinc, magnesium, vitamin E and all trace minerals. To determine your requirement for these, consider receiving some council. Additionally, the thyroid requires iodine. The following is explained for ease of independent use:

1. **Iodine** Due to the compound of iodine having a tendency to be a toxin, I suggest the dose be derived two different ways only:

   1) by consuming whole foods naturally rich in iodine / consume to enjoyment

   2) application of iodine topically.

   To introduce iodine topically, purchase a medical grade iodine tincture and follow the directions below. You may be already familiar with this tincture form of iodine because it has been used for decades to apply to cuts and bleeding rashes and sores in an effort to sterilize and optimize topical healing. At one time it may even have been included in first-aid kits. It is easily sourced at a local pharmacy. Apply the iodine in the following manner:

- Preparing the skin. Firstly, the skin needs to have been moisture-softened (by way of a bath, shower, or sponge-bath). The best areas to apply it are on parts of the body where there is fat, and where the skin is least likely to be tough from daily exposure. Good areas of skin for application is belly, buttocks, or inside thighs. *Note: Never apply the iodine to dry skin. Discomfort and irritation will happen if the skin is not well moistened before application.*

- The dose suggested is a few drops which will leave a bright orange stain on your skin.

- Apply only once in a 24-hour period. Re-apply only after the stain you created is fully gone. This can happen between 24 hours and five days. In this way, the iodine will be absorbed for use by the thyroid through the skin, in the exact amount needed, at the exact time of day it needs it most. This is, in my opinion, the safest and preferred way to receive this essential compound.

2. **Selenium.** This mineral is present in a healthy thyroid in a high concentration – the thyroid is the only place in our body that selenium is actually stored. As a result of the absence of it in our soils and modern farm cropping, I suggest that it be supplemented on a regular basis. One natural source that is highly nutritional is the Brazil nut.

3. **Sea Vegetables**. These are nori, kelp, kombu, wakame, and hiziki. I use these in the following way:

   - Nori I like to eat as a snack and "as is"; it's the wrapper used for the savory rolls featured in Japanese cuisine.

   - Kelp, wakame, and hiziki are easily consumed in flake-form that can be sprinkled as a condiment.

   - Kombu, I include in my rice cooker so the rice dish is filled with the sea nutrient. I will also put it in my slow cooker when I am making soups and stews.

4. **Raw Sea Salt.** Use a natural, unprocessed salt product. My personal favorites are Himalayan Pink Salt, Redmond's Real Salt, and Celtic Sea Salt. Each salt product is known to have unique properties that support many aspects of health in general, and the thyroid gland specifically.

5. **Certain Fruits**. Cranberries, especially the Cape Cod variety, are said to be one of the richest land-plant sources of iodine, primarily because they are grown close to the ocean. Pomegranate is especially high in both Vitamin C and fiber, along with both quercetin and bioflavonoids. Other fruits, especially the skin (organic only), contain ascorbic acid and/or nutrients that are important to healing and detoxification.

6. **Other Recommended Whole Foods.** The following foods are known to be a significant source of iodine or nutrients that support the thyroid gland: spinach, dark chocolate, eggs, seafood, prunes, potatoes, corn, and lima beans.

Nourishment for Your Body to Compensate for Missing Essential Thyroid Secretions

When thyroid glandular secretions are either not happening or impaired in any way, the entire body can become impaired and weakened. How do we feed the body with the concentrated nutrients that will help compensate for the missing thyroid secretions?

Below, I suggest some supportive nutrients that are amongst those most recommended when providing targeted physical support. Though the thyroid gland plays a role in almost every cell and organ function, the major systems that I am always guided to focus on are the thyroid itself, and the heart, kidney, and brain.

Special Note: The quality, formulation and suggested dosage of these items will vary from supplier to supplier. For the specifics on determining a dose that is best for you personally, or for a recommendation of the effectiveness of one product over another, I suggest you either have a personalized program created for you or learn how to be effective at energy testing yourself.

- <u>Among the most effective supplements and nutrients</u>: magnesium, calcium, vitamin E, selenium, omega 3/6/9, all vitamin B's – particularly vitamin B5 and B12, evening primrose, turmeric, ginger, nettle, licorice, cranberry, pomegranate, nori, sea vegetables, raw sea salt.

- <u>Among the most effective herbs:</u> Gypsywort, Siberian and Indian Ginseng, Artemisia, curcumin, cayenne, bugle, red clover, elderberry, bacopa, Ashwagandha, cat's claw, bladderwrack, black walnut, chlorophyll, nettle, spirulina, algae, kelp, kombu.
- <u>Among the most effective suggested compounds and tonics are</u>: colloidal silver
- <u>Others</u>:
  - Homeopathic remedies are signatures of innate communication. These are extremely effective.
  - As it is nearly always important to support the Adrenal Gland at the same time as the thyroid gland, Vitamin B5 should be included as a priority in the supplemental nutrients.
  - Though availability and consistent quality can be a challenge, other helpful products are those that contain compounded secretions of the thyroid gland and the adrenal gland. These can be available by way of medical care.

Special Note: It is important not to consume every one of the listed items. Each person has an individual requirement and one should consider using only the most effective. There is the potential for significant incompatibility and allergic reaction.

Chapter Nine:

CARE – Evolution & Recalibration

W e are in the process a transformation – a great collective opportunity is beckoning humanity, and everything that has come before us in history has brought us to this time. Does it look pretty or feel pleasant? Nope, it is showing itself as a struggle in the current pressures of the world and in many factions of society. It is presenting itself in the our politics, along with the signs of environmental collapse, threats of war, and epidemics, inside the civil unrest, racism and hatred. But that is just one perspective. With that perspective in mind, we just might not make it.

Thankfully, there is another perspective. In this other perspective, the familiar is fast disappearing and we now live in a world filled with daily newness. We are at a crossroad, and crossroads are where great transformations emerge. This pressure is inviting humanity into a new world, with a new way of being, and people everywhere have begun to embrace it. In this perspective, people and leaders are stepping up and calling for change. Many are expanding their consciousness and waking up to what is possible. People are attempting to find their own voice and are working actively to respect the voice of others. It is starting. People are choosing to heal.

The butterfly is a great symbol of transformation. As it struggles and fights to get out of the chrysalis, this struggle pumps blood into the wings that will make it perfectly fit to take flight. Without the struggle, the butterfly would never build its capacity to use its wings. Humanity is in a struggle of this nature.

I believe that the epidemic of thyroid gland dysfunction is symbolic of the dark night before the dawn. It is symbolic of us collectively trying to find our voice and the pressure for us to evolve to our next step in our human evolution. While many factors are actively having impact on the thyroid gland and its role in our health and wellness, the emergence of activity in two new lobes (petals of the flower) with the new colour teal, it has the vibration of perfect support. It is as if, in this new vibration, we are seeing the melding in partnership of the heart and the thyroid gland so as to find a new voice of compassion and love. By joining together in the harmony of this vibrant new voice, we will undeniably unite our talents, gifts, potentials, passions, and purposes to create and collaborate Happy is the thyroid as a flower in full bloom!

What exactly is being expected of us? Firstly, we cannot know what we don't know. Secondly, trust and patience are in order. Thirdly, that our voice, our expression and our capacity for love and compassion, is being expanded to have us co-create this new world based on deepening capacities to live consciously. This new earth will not happen overnight; we have work before we sleep. And, if this is the *truth and the way,* it is big, and every one of us here on Earth is in it together. Genuine connection, collaboration, and cooperation will be key.

Gregg Braden's book, *Human By Design,* and Kryon Book Fourteen titled *The New Human: The Evolution of*

Humanity, reference this process we are in. These current time thought leaders are ultimately here to share their insights and to guide us. They have helped me to make sense of some of what I have been shown. I believe, through their sharing scientific developments, truths, and beliefs – and by our sharing their discoveries – we will find our way as individuals, and as a collective, as painlessly as possible. A renewed and beautiful world is dawning.

Following, are two guided processes that can be done regularly to assist in the re-calibration process that is currently underway. Through these processes we can enhance the thyroid energies, expand the vibrancy of voice, and create greater ease in being ready, daily, for all that is unfolding.

COMFORTING SOUND BATH

- Step 1 – Prepare and set-up. Plan to ensure privacy for a minimum of 30 minutes.

  Get comfortable in the option of one of two spaces: either directly in a nature setting where you can be relaxed in a chair or chaise, or with headphones on and listening to a recording of the sounds of nature in your private space of home or office.

- Step 2 – Loosen your head and neck by doing a few neck rolls. Straighten your spine, drop the shoulders and tuck your chin slightly to create a neutral hanging position. This is important because it puts the thyroid gland in a calm space.

- Step 3 – As you are present in the sounds of nature, natural or recorded, enter into a feeling of appreciation or gratitude. Some will choose to think of people and things that place them in that space, and others will find it arrives on their very breath – whatever works for you is absolutely perfect.

- Step 4 – Feel your throat and the thyroid location on your body. Imagine all those pure simple sounds are speaking directly to your thyroid gland. Feel it as if your thyroid is being serenaded by the healing sounds of nature. As a sound comes to greet the thyroid, allow it to pass from the front through to the back of your neck. An endless horizontal line of flow is created.

- Step 5 – Breathing comfortably, remain in this place for the time you have available. As mentioned in set-up: ideally 30 minutes or more.

HAAAAAAA SOUND EXERCISE.

This can be done anywhere at any time, for a minute, or two, or ten, according to your availability and desire. It involves the following:

- Step 1 – Stand grounded, with feet shoulder-width apart with gentle knees, or you can sit cross-legged as a yogi if that is preferable. Place your hands comfortably by your side or in a prayer position. Feel the body quiet and calm.

- Step 2 – Breathe in deeply, and as you do, open your mouth as wide as you can. On the exhale, add to your breath an audible "haaaaaaa" sound. Empty your breath fully and repeat. *You may find that you need to cough as the muscles relax in the area – this is normal.*

- Though a bit of a showstopper done in public, this exercise is a great habit to get into as a daily practice because of the multiple benefits to the thyroid gland. Also, it stimulates the production of oxytocin. Oxytocin is known as the "cuddle hormone"and it plays a key role in our ability to interact socially and bond.

To Our Future

We are living in an incredible time here on Earth. I believe that like I know that I did, we have all made the choice to be here, and in that we have made a commitment to work through the opportunities that are being presented to us. I believe that we will always continue to have choices. Will you make the choice to accept that we are each now being given the option to *be* empowered in a new way – a way like never been before? Can you accept that we are being supported to choose to journey an illuminated path that is uncommon to any previous experience had by our civilization here on Earth?

By our care, and through our work as an intuitive (because we are all intuitives), we exercise the muscle that is our openness to receive guidance, and we trust in what we are given and shown.

You and I are never alone. Perhaps because I was born with this gift and ability, I have the confidence to tread where many may not. I have been shown that it is up to people like me and you to be examples and to show the way forward. I'm invested in you.

Let's recap.

Change: While it can feel challenging – overwhelming at times – and cause a sense of losing control, there is nothing we can do to stop change. The thyroid gland will continue to react to change. It is up to us to embrace change and care for our thyroid gland. The "pressures" from change – the opportunities to grow – have dictated the course of biological life through the evolution from bacteria, to single cells, to communities of cells, to multicellular plants and animals, to perhaps the most complex, magnificent organism on the planet today: the human body. Now, the pressures of change are calling humanity to grow and expand again. We are all a part of this magnificence. We can participate in the opportunities that are being presented to us by making wise choices.

Choice: Our power lies in acceptance. We can choose to resist change, but that choice is like swimming upstream. Resistance in itself is exhausting, makes us ill and stresses our thyroid in addition to all parts of the body, mind, and spirit. In our repertoire of strategies of resistance, we can always choose to *grab onto rocks while being swept downstream in a river*. However, if we hang onto rocks, we are sure to miss out on the newness of what is downstream. Amazing events await us and carry us forward, as long as we agree to let go. In this emerging world, it is downstream where you will find your perfect health, abundance, freedom, and joy.

Care: I equate care to love. Loving yourself involves taking care of your thyroid so that you can attain the optimal health and vitality you totally deserve. The CARE program in this book included:

- **Cleansing & Clearing**: Letting go and clearing everything that is interfering with thyroid health and blocking the flow of your life. Vitality is ours when we remove all (physical, emotional) that no longer serves.

- **Acceptance, Alignment, Balance & Movement**: Within acceptance is peace. Move your body so that it can align and balance. Get up and dance, and practice acceptance, appreciation, and gratitude each and every day.

- **Replenishing & Nourishing:** Your thyroid needs quality nourishment for its growth and renewal. Take action to nourish your body and your thyroid with poignant nutrition.
- **Evolution & Re calibration:** Humanity is at the cusp of a great transformation. Embrace your part and purpose in this process. The future is ours!

Celebration: I celebrate you and invite you to consider all the possibilities and potential that lies ahead. BE fully aware of the blessing we are receiving by being here at this time. We are in it to love!

I trust you understand that, in the illness and upset around your thyroid, there is both an opportunity and a profound message. It has arrived in your life because you are being called. Yes, called to learn how you are to be efficacious in your choosing to heal, stabilize and renew. You and I are being given the opportunity to connect in new ways and to serve and care! Further, I ask you to consider that new and powerful upgrades are happening all the time and that this will be ongoing. Illness has arrived, not with the intention to weaken or destroy you, but to be a tool of motivation so that you will ultimately be encouraged to expand beyond what is known and tangible. Please hold faith and trust in your divinity. It has always been intended that humanity would ultimately have a beautiful time of "the time" that is here and now. I have no doubt that we are to be a new human.

Acknowledgments
With Heartfelt Gratitude

You know how you don't know what you don't know? Well, I had no idea of what went into writing a book. Wow! I want to thank the family of people who supported me in every way so that I would complete on my commitment to share through this written word.

Richard Schultz – My friend who has long been an iconic and steadfast sounding board, a voice of encouragement, a great coach and teacher. *Thank you for writing the foreword of this book, and for being here with me for it all – the journey, this work and the creation.*

Marie Beswick-Arthur – The slogan of her business is "writing to change the world." *She is a brilliant and compassionate person without whose support and expertise I could not have sprinted across the finish line of writing this book.*

David Newans – *For including me along his journey with health. For being a text-book example to learn and glean from. I will always look forward to hearing your laughter! Am grateful to see the brilliance of your ever-shining light.*

Brenda Hanna – My interpreter of all things beautiful. *Thank you for the years of our time together and for always coming through for me. For the artistic base of the cover of this book.*

Dr. Angela Lauria – Who got me in gear and showed me the way.

David Hancock and the Morgan James Publishing team – thank you for helping me bring this book to print.

Skylar Newans – I met her when she was seven and have watched her grow into a bright and beautiful woman. *Your presence in my life and my work brings me such happiness. Thank you for making a difference in my world.*

My grandchildren: Tayla, Tenley, and Benton – When you were a wee toddler, precious Tayla you named me your LaLa. I am filled with joy to be here with you and your sister and brother! Individually and together, you are each my greatest joy! *Thank you for coming to play with your LaLa.* And to Jaden – thank you for letting me choose you to be mine too!

My sons: James and Richard – Your arrival brought richness to my life in the most unexpected and profound ways. *Thank you for choosing me to be your Mum! Thank you for all you have taught me and, in advance for all you will continue to teach me.*

Vernon and Anne: My parents – For their perfect imperfection. *I miss you.*

My sisters and brother – For being my mirror, and for the unforgettable life lessons.

Dorothy Corney – My hero. My role model. I now give in the spirit of all you gave to me. *You always knew just the right things to say. Gone from this life, you are always with me. I look forward to when next we will have tea.*

Lee Bussard – You have been long gone from this world. but you are never, ever forgotten.

Anja and Don Cawthorne – Living examples of how love is work made manifest. *For the past years of constant connection, and for how you steadfastly model simplicity and magnificence.*

Lee Carroll and Kryon – *Your very appearance and presence have made it that, in recent years, I would be encouraged and energized when I was discouraged and depleted. And that I could understand when I was disillusioned and confused. Thank you from ALL of me from every lifetime and through all of time.*

Marilyn Harper and Adironnda – *Your contribution of wisdom for this time, your humour and heart are making this world a better place. I love hearing your sweet voice! Your open arms and embrace has meant the world to me. Thank you for Being!*

Blaine Michalsky – My adorable life partner and best friend. *You cuddle me when I need to be held and are my always loving hand to hold. Thank you for picking me! Thank you for BE-ing!*

And finally,

Thank You to both the Divine and to those from the realm not visible here now, who counsel me. You are my light and my way. Your unfailing presence for the whole of my life has made it that I am never ever alone – truly awesome that you are always only a mere thought away. I have not enough words to tell you how honoured I am to BE an incarnated extension of your collective commitment to loving and caring for humanity.

Thank You!

Dear One,

If you have arrived at this place in this book, it is 100% because you had either been curious, or you are a Seeker. I am thrilled that I could be here for you and that I am here with you now. Thank you for this honour!

Are you looking for further assistance with your thyroid gland health or to receive other health information, personalized insight and care? Please reach out to connect by visiting **www.vannette.ca** and by emailing me at **vannettek@outlook.com**. I would love to have you join me in one of my offerings so that I may assist your further!

The following are among my offerings:

- Study Group – Featuring the CARE System discussed in chapters 6,7,8 and 9 of this book. Receive the benefit of engaging directly with myself for counsel and connecting with like-minded others.

- One-on-One Coaching – Receive the benefits of one-on-one support and assistance with a focus on healing, health and personalized insights.
- Retreats – Several times a year in nature settings, my retreats provide opportunities to connect in community and to receive real healthcare, personalized protocols and individualized strategies to cleanse and receive healing.
- Access to quality healing products. I have personally chosen health products which I recommend because of their quality, harmony and resonance. These are available for purchase through my office and can be shipped via standard shipping or drop-shipping throughout both Canada and the USA.

May joy and peace surround you,
Contentment latch your door
And happiness be with you now,
And bless you evermore.
– Irish Blessing

Vannette

About the Author

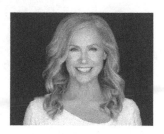

Vannette Keast is an Intuitive, an Empath, and Healer. Born with a servant's heart, she's always heard messages, had visions, and has innately known information designed to assist us all in this lifetime here on Earth. Her first memory of this life is of being on the other side and asked if she would return to Earth for this time. Dedicated to her practice, a career spanning more than two decades, she has had the distinct honour to be part of many health success stories and miracles – more than six hundred people a year, worldwide, have engaged to become clients.

Outside her thriving practice based in Red Deer, Alberta, Canada, she shares her home with the love of her life, Blaine; Vannette spends time daily in nature, loves travel adventures, and enjoys playtime with granddaughters Tayla Rose and Tenley Grace, and grandsons Benton and Jaden.

CPSIA information can be obtained
at www.ICGtesting.com
Printed in the USA
LVHW012254300820
664598LV00002B/411

9 781642 798654